COMPLETE GUIDE TO UNDERSTANDING CARPAL TUNNEL RELEASE

Comprehensive Manual On In-Depth Techniques, Symptoms, Treatments, And Recovery For Optimal Hand Health

KLEIN HOYLE

Disclaimer

The content in this book is based on the author's expertise and comprehension of the topic. The author has no affiliation or link with any corporation, business, or person. This book is meant to give general information and educational material only, and it should not be interpreted as professional medical advice. Always seek the advice of a skilled healthcare expert if you have any queries about medical issues or treatments. The author and publisher expressly disclaim any responsibility resulting directly or indirectly from the use or use of the information included in this book.

Table of Contents

ABOUT THIS BOOK

The "Complete Guide to Understanding Carpal Tunnel Release" is an essential resource for anybody dealing with the difficulties of carpal tunnel syndrome (CTS) or considering carpal tunnel release surgery. This extensive booklet digs into the complexities of CTS, from basic ideas to surgical surgery and long-term care techniques.

Chapter 1 of the book delves further into carpal tunnel syndrome, explaining its foundations, symptoms, and risk factors. Understanding the significance of early diagnosis and treatment lays the groundwork for informed decision-making, making this introductory chapter required reading for both patients and healthcare providers.

In Chapter 2, readers delve further into the anatomy of the wrist and carpal tunnel, learning about the various structures and roles involved. Understanding the basic mechanics of CTS development allows people to better understand the reasons for treatment options covered later in the book.

Chapter 3 focuses on non-surgical therapy alternatives, providing a comprehensive approach to symptom management. Lifestyle changes, physical therapy exercises, and pharmaceutical methods provide readers with realistic solutions for reducing pain and improving quality of life.

For individuals contemplating surgical intervention, Chapter 4 offers vital advice on preparation and risk assessment. From the first consultation to post-operative care, this section provides patients with the information they need to confidently navigate the surgical path.

Chapter 5 delves into the complexities of carpal tunnel release surgery, examining several procedures and their benefits. By diving into surgical intricacies and issues, readers may make more educated choices with their healthcare providers.

Chapter 6 presents a step-by-step overview of the surgical technique, demystifying it and allaying fears. Detailed details of anesthetic alternatives, incision procedures, and post-operative care standards ensure that readers are well-prepared for what lies ahead.

After surgery, Chapter 7 walks readers through the healing and rehabilitation process. Practical pain management suggestions and exercises for recovering wrist functioning allow people to actively engage in their recovery process.

In Chapter 8, the book digs into the possible dangers and difficulties of carpal tunnel release surgery, to raise awareness and prepare readers. By addressing issues front on, readers may face surgery with a healthy mindset and reasonable expectations.

Long-term management techniques take priority in Chapter 9, emphasizing the necessity of continuous monitoring and preventative actions. Individuals may reduce the chance of recurrence and improve their hand health by making lifestyle changes and paying attention to their bodies.

Finally, Chapter 10 takes a comprehensive approach to lifestyle changes and preventative interventions, highlighting the need for proactive self-care. From ergonomic office arrangements to early symptom assessment, this section teaches readers how to take proactive control of their hand health.

In summary, "Complete Guide to Understanding Carpal Tunnel Release" is more than just instructional literature; it serves as a beacon of empowerment and enlightenment for anyone navigating the complexity of carpal tunnel syndrome and its therapeutic terrain.

CHAPTER 1
Introduction To Carpal Tunnel Syndrome

Understanding The Basics Of Carpal Tunnel Syndrome

Carpal tunnel syndrome (CTS) is a widespread disorder affecting the hands and wrists. To further grasp it, let's look at the anatomy of the wrist. The carpal tunnel is a tiny corridor produced by your wrist's bones and ligaments. The median nerve passes through this tunnel, controlling sensation and movement in the thumb and first three fingers.

Carpal tunnel syndrome symptoms are caused when the median nerve is pinched or crushed. This compression may develop for a variety of causes, including repeated hand motions, wrist injuries, or medical diseases such as arthritis.

Recognize The Symptoms And Risk Factors

Recognizing the symptoms of carpal tunnel syndrome is critical for proper treatment. The most common symptoms are numbness, tingling, and discomfort in the hands and fingers, especially at night. Some people may have weakness in their afflicted hand, making it difficult to hold things or do fine motor skills.

Several factors may increase the likelihood of getting carpal tunnel syndrome. These include repetitive hand motions like typing or assembly line jobs, as well as diseases including obesity, diabetes, and thyroid issues. Women are also more susceptible to CTS, particularly after pregnancy and menopause.

Importance Of Early Detection And Treatment

Early identification of carpal tunnel syndrome is critical to preventing it from progressing and causing lasting nerve damage.

Ignoring symptoms or delaying treatment may result in chronic hand and wrist disorders that impair everyday activities and quality of life.

Carpal tunnel syndrome may be treated conservatively with wrist splinting, medicines, and physical therapy, or more invasively with corticosteroid injections and surgery. Treatment is determined by the severity of the symptoms and other variables unique to each patient.

Overview Of Carpal Tunnel Release Surgery

Carpal tunnel release surgery is a frequent operation used to relieve pressure on the median nerve and improve symptoms of carpal tunnel syndrome. During the procedure, the physician creates an incision in the palm or wrist and slices the ligament that forms the roof of the carpal tunnel. This expands the tunnel and relieves pressure on the median nerve, hence reducing symptoms.

There are two techniques for carpal tunnel release surgery: open surgery and endoscopic surgery. Open surgery involves making a wider incision in the palm to have direct access to the carpal tunnel. Endoscopic surgery, on the other hand, employs a tiny camera and specialized equipment introduced via small incisions to see and loosen the ligament.

Both procedures strive for the same goal: to relieve pressure on the median nerve and improve carpal tunnel syndrome symptoms. Patient desire, physician competence, and anatomical considerations all play a role in determining whether to do open or endoscopic surgery.

Understanding the foundations of carpal tunnel syndrome, identifying its symptoms and risk factors, and emphasizing the need for early identification and treatment are critical for successfully treating this illness.

CHAPTER 2

Anatomy Of The Wrist And Carpal Tunnel

Exploring The Structure Of The Wrist

Understanding the anatomy of the wrist is critical to understanding carpal tunnel release. The wrist is a complicated joint made up of many bones, ligaments, tendons, and nerves. The carpal tunnel—a tiny conduit produced by the carpal bones and the transverse carpal ligament—is at the heart of this complex network. This tunnel connects various structures, including the median nerve and the flexor tendons that control finger movement.

Consider the wrist to be a busy junction where nerves and tendons pass via a narrow corridor. Any interruption in this channel may cause pain, numbness, and weakness, which are the characteristics of carpal tunnel syndrome.

Understanding the architecture of the wrist allows us to better understand the issues that this disease presents as well as the reasoning for carpal tunnel release.

Function Of The Carpal Tunnel

The carpal tunnel is essential for allowing smooth hand motions. It serves as a protective sheath, keeping the median nerve and flexor tendons secure from external compression or damage. During wrist and finger flexion tasks, such as typing or grasping things, the carpal tunnel provides an ideal environment for nerve and tendon activity.

Think of the carpal tunnel as a subway tunnel. Nerves and tendons pass through the carpal tunnel in the same way as trains do, allowing for smooth communication between the brain and hand muscles. However, when the tunnel gets clogged owing to inflammation or edema, this flow may be impeded, resulting in carpal tunnel syndrome-like sensations.

Nerves And Tendons In The Wrist

The wrist contains a network of nerves and tendons that are essential for hand motion. Among these structures, the median nerve gets the spotlight. The median nerve originates in the neck's brachial plexus and goes down the arm to the carpal tunnel, where it supplies feeling to the thumb, index finger, middle finger, and part of the ring finger. Along with the median nerve, flexor tendons responsible for finger bending pass through the carpal tunnel.

Imagine the wrist as a lively bazaar, with nerves and tendons moving about like consumers on a mission. Each nerve impulse and tendon movement is carefully coordinated to guarantee proper hand function. However, when there is congestion inside the carpal tunnel, the smooth passage of these important components is disturbed, causing pain and malfunction.

How Carpal Tunnel Syndrome Develops

Carpal tunnel syndrome results from a combination of causes, including anatomical predisposition, repeated hand motions, and underlying medical disorders. The tight constraints of the carpal tunnel render it prone to compression, especially when exposed to prolonged or recurrent wrist-straining exercises.

Consider a river moving through a tight canyon. Under normal circumstances, the water flows freely, nourishing the surrounding environment. However, as debris accumulates or the channel narrows, the flow becomes blocked, resulting in stagnation and overflow. Similarly, with carpal tunnel syndrome, repeated hand motions or illnesses such as arthritis may induce swelling or inflammation, compressing the median nerve and producing symptoms such as numbness, tingling, and weakness.

Understanding the underlying processes of carpal tunnel syndrome is critical for successful management and therapy. By understanding the relationship between anatomy, function, and pathology, healthcare clinicians may customize therapies like carpal tunnel release to relieve symptoms and restore hand function.

CHAPTER 3

Non-Surgical Treatment Options

Lifestyle Adjustments To Relieve Symptoms

Lifestyle adjustments may help alleviate the symptoms of carpal tunnel syndrome. These modifications often include changing daily tasks to alleviate wrist and hand discomfort. Simple changes, such as taking frequent pauses from repetitive jobs, maintaining correct posture, and avoiding activities that exacerbate symptoms, may make a significant impact.

Ergonomics is an important consideration when making lifestyle modifications. This entails organizing your desk to encourage good posture and prevent strain on your wrists and hands. For example, altering the height and angle of your computer keyboard and mouse may assist relieve pressure on the median nerve, which travels through the carpal tunnel in your wrist.

Another important lifestyle modification is maintaining your weight and general health. Excess weight might increase pressure on the median nerve, exacerbating CTS symptoms. Maintaining a healthy weight via food and exercise may help lower blood pressure and relieve symptoms.

Additionally, maintaining proper wrist and hand posture throughout the day might assist avoid additional aggravation of the median nerve. This might involve maintaining your wrists in a neutral posture when typing or using tools, rather than bending them at sharp angles.

Lifestyle improvements such as ergonomic adjustments, weight control, and appropriate posture may help alleviate the symptoms of carpal tunnel syndrome.

Making these easy changes may minimize stress on the median nerve and enhance your overall quality of life.

Physical Therapy Activities To Improve Wrist Mobility

Physical therapy exercises may be a useful non-surgical treatment for carpal tunnel syndrome. These exercises are intended to enhance wrist mobility, strengthen hand and forearm muscles, and alleviate the discomfort and inflammation associated with carpal tunnel syndrome.

Wrist flexor and extensor stretches are frequent physical therapy exercises for chronic tension syndrome. These exercises enhance wrist flexibility and range of motion, which reduces strain on the median nerve. Wrist flexion and extension exercises are examples of these stretches, in which you gently bend your wrist forward and backward while holding each stretch for a few seconds.

Nerve gliding, also known as neural mobilization, is another useful activity. This entails mild motions that assist mobilize the median nerve, so relieving compression, and enhancing nerve function. Nerve gliding activities for CTS include wrist circles and tendon glides, which stretch and mobilize the median nerve via its course in the wrist.

Exercises that strengthen the muscles of the hand and forearm may also help relieve CTS symptoms. These exercises usually include utilizing resistance bands or hand weights to strengthen the muscles that support the wrist and hands. Examples include wrist curls, grip workouts, and finger extensions.

In addition to these particular exercises, physical therapists may propose activities that improve general posture and body mechanics, hence reducing pressure on the wrists and hands.

Physical therapy exercises for wrist mobility may be a useful non-surgical treatment for carpal tunnel syndrome. Individuals with CTS may benefit from these exercises because they enhance flexibility, strength, and general function in the wrist and hand.

Splinting And Ergonomic Modifications

Splinting and ergonomic changes are effective non-surgical treatments for carpal tunnel syndrome. These procedures relieve pain, numbness, and tingling by lowering pressure on the median nerve in the wrist.

Splinting is wearing a brace or splint on the wrist to maintain it in a neutral posture, hence reducing compression on the median nerve. Splints may relieve symptoms and prevent additional stimulation of the median nerve during activities that aggravate CTS symptoms by immobilizing the wrist in this posture.

Ergonomic changes are designed to alleviate wrist and hand strain by improving the workstation and everyday activities.

This may include altering the height and angle of the computer keyboard and mouse, employing ergonomic tools and equipment, and taking frequent pauses from repetitive work to relax and extend the hands and wrists.

In addition to splinting and ergonomic adaptations, further changes to regular routines may be suggested. Individuals suffering from CTS, for example, may be advised to avoid occupations that demand repeated wrist motions or hard grasping, since these might aggravate their symptoms.

Overall, splinting and ergonomic changes are significant aspects of non-surgical carpal tunnel syndrome therapy. These therapies, which reduce pressure on the median nerve and promote appropriate wrist and hand posture, may assist persons with CTS relieve symptoms and enhance their overall quality of life.

Medications For Pain Treatment

Carpal tunnel syndrome (CTS) discomfort may be effectively managed non-surgically with medications. These drugs help people with CTS by lowering inflammation, and discomfort, and increasing overall comfort.

Nonsteroidal anti-inflammatory medicines (NSAIDs), such as ibuprofen and naproxen, may help decrease inflammation and discomfort caused by CTS. These drugs are available over the counter and may help with mild to moderate symptoms.

In rare circumstances, corticosteroid injections may be used to relieve inflammation and discomfort in the wrist. These injections are given directly into the carpal tunnel, which may offer brief relief from discomfort.

Topical treatments like lidocaine patches or lotions may also be used to numb the wrist and relieve discomfort caused by CTS. These drugs are administered directly to the skin and may give localized relief from pain.

It is critical to speak with a healthcare expert before beginning any pharmaceutical regimen for CTS, as they can advise on the proper dose and any adverse effects.

Medicines may be an effective nonsurgical therapy option for carpal tunnel syndrome discomfort. These drugs help enhance CTS patients' overall comfort and quality of life by lowering inflammation and discomfort.

CHAPTER 4

Preparing For Carpal Tunnel Release Surgery

Consult With A Healthcare Professional

Before having carpal tunnel release surgery, you should contact a healthcare expert, usually a hand surgeon or an orthopedic specialist. This consultation is an important stage in the process since it allows the healthcare practitioner to evaluate your symptoms, medical history, and general health to decide if surgery is the best option.

During the consultation, your doctor will inquire about your symptoms, such as discomfort, numbness, and weakness in your hands and fingers. They may also question about past therapies you have tried and their efficacy.

This information allows them to assess the severity of your problem and determine if surgery is required.

In addition to discussing your symptoms, your doctor will do a physical examination to determine the strength, feeling, and movement of your hand and fingers. They may also do other tests, such as Tinel's sign and Phalen's test, to assess your condition.

Based on the information acquired during the consultation and examination, your healthcare practitioner will explain the possible advantages and risks of carpal tunnel release surgery to you. They will answer any issues or questions you may have and provide suggestions based on your specific situation.

Finally, the consultation allows you and your healthcare professional to work together on a treatment plan that is tailored to your specific objectives and preferences. If all parties agree that surgery is the best choice, you will go on to the following stages in preparation for the operation.

Diagnostic Tests To Confirm The Diagnosis

Following the first appointment, your healthcare professional may suggest diagnostic testing to confirm the diagnosis of carpal tunnel syndrome and determine its severity. These tests serve to determine that surgery is suitable and give useful information to guide the surgical procedure.

Carpal tunnel syndrome is often diagnosed with electromyography (EMG) and nerve conduction studies (NCS). EMG includes inserting tiny needles into the muscles of the hand and forearm to monitor electrical activity and evaluate nerve function. NCS involves sending tiny electrical shocks to the nerves in the hand and evaluating the speed and intensity of the resultant nerve signals.

In addition, your healthcare practitioner may perform imaging studies, such as X-rays or ultrasounds, to assess the wrist structures and rule out other possible reasons for your symptoms.

These diagnostic tests allow your healthcare professional to confirm the diagnosis of carpal tunnel syndrome, assess the degree of nerve compression, and design the best surgical treatment. They give crucial information that helps guide decision-making and assures the best potential surgical result.

Pre-Operative Instructions And Considerations

In the days leading up to carpal tunnel release surgery, your healthcare practitioner will give you detailed pre-operative instructions to follow. These recommendations are intended to help you prepare for the treatment while reducing the chance of problems.

Medication management is a crucial factor. To lessen the risk of bleeding during surgery, your doctor may advise you to cease taking certain medicines, such as blood thinners or nonsteroidal anti-inflammatory drugs (NSAIDs), in the days leading up to the operation.

You may also be told not to eat or drink for a set amount of time before surgery, which usually begins at midnight the night before. This fasting interval helps to avoid anesthesia-related issues and assures your safety during the operation.

In addition, your healthcare professional may suggest particular exercises or stretches to do in the days preceding surgery to help preserve flexibility and strength in your hand and wrist. These exercises may also assist in reducing symptoms and enhance post-operative recovery.

Finally, your healthcare professional will discuss the surgery's details with you, such as the date, time, and place. They will answer any lingering questions or concerns you may have, ensuring that you are aware and prepared for the next procedure.

Potential Dangers And Complications

Carpal tunnel release surgery, like any other surgical operation, has risks and problems that you should be aware of before undergoing it. While the overall risk is minimal, recognizing these possible consequences will help you decide if surgery is suitable for you.

Infection at the operative site is one of the risks associated with carpal tunnel release surgery. To reduce this danger, your healthcare professional will sterilize the devices and use sterile practices throughout the treatment. They may also prescribe medications to lessen the likelihood of infection after surgery.

Another possible consequence is nerve injury, which may cause temporary or permanent alterations in feeling or movement in the hand and fingers. Nerve injury is rare, however, it may occur during the surgical operation or as a consequence of scar tissue development during the healing period.

Other risks and consequences of carpal tunnel release surgery include bleeding, blood clots, anesthesia-related allergies, and hand or wrist stiffness or paralysis. Your healthcare practitioner will thoroughly explain these risks to you and take precautions to reduce them during the surgical process.

Overall, although the risks and problems of carpal tunnel release surgery must be considered, many patients find that the advantages of discomfort relief and improved hand function exceed the dangers. By discussing these issues with your healthcare practitioner and following their advice, you can make an educated choice about whether surgery is suitable for you.

CHAPTER 5

Types Of Carpal Tunnel Release Surgery

Open Carpal Tunnel Release Procedure

Open carpal tunnel release surgery is a popular surgical treatment for treating carpal tunnel syndrome (CTS), which is characterized by numbness, tingling, and weakness in the hand and wrist. During this procedure, the surgeon creates an incision in the palm to expose the transverse carpal ligament—the band of tissue that surrounds the carpal tunnel. The surgeon then delicately slices the ligament, reducing pressure on the median nerve and eliminating CTS symptoms.

One benefit of the open carpal tunnel release treatment is that it allows for direct vision of the carpal tunnel and its surroundings, which may aid in the exact cutting of the transverse carpal ligament. Furthermore, this procedure is quite simple and has been used for many years, resulting in a well-established surgical strategy with predictable results for patients.

After cutting the ligament, sutures are used to seal the incision in the palm, and a bandage or dressing is put to cover the surgical site. Patients sometimes suffer some soreness and swelling after the treatment, but this normally goes away within a few weeks with careful care and therapy. Physical therapy may be suggested to help restore strength and range of motion in the hand and wrist.

Endoscopic Carpal Tunnel Release Technique

The endoscopic carpal tunnel release method is a less intrusive alternative to open surgery. Instead of creating a major incision in the palm, the surgeon makes one or two tiny incisions and inserts a thin, flexible tube known as an endoscope into the carpal tunnel.

The endoscope has a small camera that enables the surgeon to view within the tunnel and direct minuscule surgical tools to sever the transverse carpal ligament.

One of the key benefits of the endoscopic approach is that it requires fewer incisions and causes less tissue damage than open surgery. This may result in shorter recovery durations, less postoperative discomfort, and a decreased chance of problems like infection or scarring. Furthermore, since the incisions are smaller, there may be less apparent scarring after the procedure.

However, the endoscopic procedure requires specific training and equipment, and not all surgeons are skilled in this area. Furthermore, since the surgery is conducted using a camera and small equipment, there is a danger of harm to nearby nerves and tissues if not done correctly. Patients seeking endoscopic carpal tunnel release should consult with their surgeon to fully understand the risks and benefits.

Comparison Of Surgical Approaches

When selecting between open and endoscopic carpal tunnel release, various aspects must be addressed, including the severity of the patient's complaints, their general health and medical history, and the surgeon's experience and preference. Both procedures have been demonstrated to help treat CTS symptoms, although they vary in terms of invasiveness, recovery time, and possible consequences.

Open carpal tunnel release is a more conventional method that has been utilized for decades, while the endoscopic release is a more recent, less invasive procedure. Endoscopic release may provide shorter recovery periods and less surgical discomfort, but it may not be appropriate for all patients, especially those with complicated cases or anatomical variances.

Before making a selection, patients should consult with their surgeon about their alternatives and assess the advantages and disadvantages of each.

Finally, the purpose of surgery is to reduce CTS symptoms and enhance the patient's quality of life, and the surgical approach used should be determined by what is appropriate for the specific patient.

Factors Influencing The Choice Of Surgery

Several variables might impact the decision to have carpal tunnel release surgery, including the severity of the patient's symptoms, their medical history, and personal preferences. Patients with mild to severe symptoms of CTS may benefit from conservative therapies such as splinting, corticosteroid injections, or physical therapy before undergoing surgery.

However, if conservative therapies fail to offer significant relief or if the patient's symptoms are severe and interfere with their regular activities, surgery may be advised. When selecting between open and endoscopic carpal tunnel release, the surgeon will consider the patient's age, employment, general health, and any underlying medical issues that may influence the success of the operation.

Patients with diabetes or peripheral neuropathy, for example, may be at a greater risk of problems such as poor wound healing or nerve damage, therefore the less intrusive endoscopic method may be beneficial. Patients with broad or prominent median nerves, on the other hand, may benefit more from open carpal tunnel release since it allows for greater tissue visibility and manipulation.

The surgeon's expertise and training in each procedure may also influence the decision-making process. Patients should feel free to share their concerns and wishes with their surgeon, as well as ask questions regarding the risks, advantages, and predicted results of each surgical option.

CHAPTER 6

Surgical Procedure Step-By-Step

Anesthesia Options For Carpal Tunnel Release

When preparing for carpal tunnel release surgery, one critical consideration is the kind of anesthetic you will get. Your surgeon will go over numerous alternatives with you, taking into consideration things like your medical history, preferences, and the intricacy of the treatment.

Local anesthesia:

Local anesthetic is routinely utilized during carpal tunnel release surgery. It involves injecting numbing drugs directly into the wrist, essentially preventing pain impulses from reaching the brain. With local anesthetic, you will be awake throughout the procedure but will not experience any discomfort.

You may experience pressure or minor discomfort while the surgeon works, but it should not be severe.

Regional Anaesthesia:

Another alternative for carpal tunnel release is a regional anesthetic, which may be administered via a wrist or axillary block. This form of anesthesia numbs a greater region than local anesthesia, allowing for more widespread pain relief. Wrist blocks include injecting anesthetic around the nerves that give a feeling to the wrist, hand, and fingers. An axillary block targets nerves in the armpit region. With regional anesthetic, you will most likely be awake throughout the procedure, but you will not experience any discomfort in the operational area.

General anesthesia:

In other circumstances, general anesthetic may be preferable, particularly if you are concerned about being awake throughout the treatment or if the surgery is complicated. General anesthesia causes unconsciousness, so you will be sleeping during the operation with no discomfort or knowledge of the process. It is delivered by intravenous drugs and breathing agents, and you will be carefully watched by an anesthesiologist during the procedure.

Incision Location And Tissue Exposure

After the anesthetic wears off, your surgeon will make an incision in the palm of your hand. The exact site of the incision may differ based on the surgeon's choice, the severity of your carpal tunnel syndrome, and any prior procedures in the region.

Palm incision:

The most frequent method for carpal tunnel release includes creating a tiny incision in the palm, usually between the base of the palm and the wrist crease. This permits the surgeon to reach the transverse carpal ligament and accomplish the release without inflicting too much stress on the surrounding tissues.

Endoscopic Technique:

In certain situations, your surgeon may choose an endoscopic method, which includes inserting a small camera and specialized tools via one or more small incisions. This approach allows for smaller incisions and perhaps quicker healing periods. The camera enables the surgeon to see the interior tissues of the wrist and guide the tools precisely.

Tissue Exposure:

After making the incision, the surgeon meticulously dissects through the layers of tissue to reveal the transverse carpal ligament, a band of tissue that compresses the median nerve in carpal tunnel syndrome. During this stage, special care is required not to damage nerves, blood vessels, or tendons.

The objective is to provide appropriate exposure for the ligament while limiting harm to neighboring tissues.

Release Of The Transverse Carpal Ligament

After exposing the transverse carpal ligament, the next step is to release it to alleviate pressure on the medial nerve. The release may be performed using a variety of procedures, depending on the surgeon's choice and the individual anatomy of the patient.

Open Release:

In an open carpal tunnel release, the surgeon cuts along the length of the transverse carpal ligament using a scalpel or surgical scissors. This successfully expands the carpal tunnel while relieving strain on the median nerve. Care is made to ensure that the ligament is completely released while minimizing injury to the surrounding tissues.

Endoscopic Release:

A surgeon performs an endoscopic carpal tunnel release by inserting specialized equipment via tiny incisions to view and sever the transverse carpal ligament. The camera magnifies the ligament and adjacent structures, enabling for accurate incisions while causing minimum disturbance to neighboring tissues.

Partial Release:

In certain circumstances, a partial relaxation of the transverse carpal ligament may be enough to alleviate symptoms. This entails releasing a piece of the ligament to increase room inside the carpal tunnel without totally cutting it. Partial release may be beneficial for those with fewer symptoms or specific anatomical concerns.

Closure And Postoperative Care Instructions

Once the transverse carpal ligament has been loosened, the incision is carefully closed with sutures or surgical staples. To protect the wound during the first few days after healing, a sterile dressing is usually used. Your surgeon will give you specific instructions for caring for the incision and controlling discomfort in the days and weeks after surgery.

Hand Elevation with Ice:

To decrease swelling and pain, keep your hand raised above heart level as much as possible in the first few days after surgery. Ice packs may also assist in reducing swelling and discomfort in the surgery region. Make sure you follow your surgeon's instructions regarding icing frequency and duration.

Hand Exercises:

As your hand recovers, your surgeon may suggest mild exercises to help you regain strength and movement. These exercises usually aim to progressively increase the range of motion while also strengthening the muscles of the hand and wrist. To minimize difficulties, these activities should be started carefully and without excessive intensity.

Follow-Up Appointments:

Your surgeon will arrange follow-up sessions to check on your progress and guarantee optimal healing. During these meetings, they will examine the incision site, check your range of motion and strength, and discuss any concerns or issues that may emerge. Attend all follow-up visits as planned and quickly express any changes or concerns to your surgeon.

CHAPTER 7

Recovery Process And Rehabilitation

Immediate Postoperative Care At The Hospital

Following carpal tunnel release surgery, quick post-operative care is critical to ensure a smooth recovery. When you wake up from anesthesia, your hand and wrist will most likely be put in a bandage or splint for support and protection. Your medical team will regularly monitor your vital signs to ensure that you are comfortable.

It is common to feel some pain or discomfort after surgery. Your doctor may prescribe pain relievers to alleviate any discomfort. They may also suggest elevating your hand to minimize swelling and administering cold packs to the surgery site on an as-needed basis.

During your hospital stay, your medical team will provide you with wound care recommendations, such as how to keep the incision site clean and dry to avoid infection. They will also educate you about potential consequences, such as severe bleeding or infection.

Depending on the kind of anesthetic used during the operation, you may feel groggy or drowsy afterward. It is critical to have someone accompany you home from the hospital and help you with everyday tasks as required during your early recovery phase.

Pain Management Strategies For Home

Once you're released from the hospital, controlling pain at home becomes a top focus in the early stages of rehabilitation. Your doctor may prescribe pain relievers or suggest over-the-counter remedies to help you feel better.

In addition to medicine, you may use various pain management measures at home. Applying cold packs to the surgery site at regular intervals will help decrease swelling and numb the region, giving comfort. It is critical to follow your doctor's advice for the frequency and duration of ice treatment.

Keeping your hand up above the heart might also help reduce swelling and pain. You may use pillows to prop up your hand when resting or sleeping to improve circulation and prevent fluid accumulation in the wrists.

It is critical to find a balance between rest and modest movement throughout the recuperation phase. While it is important to avoid intense activities that may strain the wrist, simple exercises and stretching as prescribed by your doctor may help prevent stiffness and aid recovery.

Gradual Return To Normal Activity And Work

As you heal, you will gradually resume regular activities and job obligations. However, use care and prevent overexertion, particularly in the early phases of recuperation.

Your doctor will advise you on when it is safe to resume particular activities depending on your personal development and the nature of your employment. In certain circumstances, you may need to alter specific duties or employ ergonomic devices to decrease wrist strain and avoid reinjury.

Listen to your body for any indicators of pain or exhaustion. Pace yourself and take pauses as required to prevent overloading your wrist.

If you are experiencing prolonged discomfort or difficulties doing chores, please visit your doctor for more information.

They may offer changes to your rehabilitation plan or extra therapies to help you recover.

Rehab Exercises For Wrist Strength And Flexibility

Rehabilitation activities are essential for recovering wrist strength and flexibility after carpal tunnel release surgery. Your doctor or physical therapist will recommend an exercise regimen suited to your specific requirements and objectives.

These exercises often aim to improve range of motion, strengthen the muscles around the wrist, and increase flexibility. They may include wrist stretches, light resistance workouts, and functional motions that simulate everyday tasks.

To enhance the efficacy of these exercises and reduce the danger of problems, they must be performed regularly and properly.

Begin cautiously, then gradually increase the intensity and length of your exercises as tolerated.

In addition to official rehabilitation activities, making modest lifestyle changes may help improve wrist health and avoid future problems. This might involve keeping excellent posture, using suitable ergonomics, and taking frequent pauses to relax and stretch during lengthy periods of exertion.

You may improve your recovery and restore full function in your wrist over time by adhering to your rehabilitation plan and being proactive about wrist care. Remember to be honest with your healthcare team about any issues or problems you have along the road, as they can provide essential support and assistance throughout your recovery.

CHAPTER 8

Possible Risks And Complications

Infection At The Surgery Site

One of the possible complications of carpal tunnel release surgery is surgical site infection. While infections are uncommon, it is important to be aware of the risk and take appropriate measures. Infection may develop when germs penetrate the wound site during or after surgery.

To reduce the danger of infection, surgeons and healthcare personnel adhere to stringent guidelines for preserving sterility during the process. This involves thoroughly handwashing, donning sterile gloves and gowns, and utilizing clean devices and drapes. Patients may also get antibiotics before, during, or after surgery to lessen the risk of infection.

After surgery, patients must follow the wound care guidelines supplied by their healthcare team. This usually entails keeping the incision site clean and dry, changing dressings as indicated, and avoiding activities that may introduce germs into the wound. Infection symptoms, such as increased pain, redness, swelling, or discharge from the incision, should be reported to your healthcare professional every once for examination and treatment.

Nerve Injury And Worsening Symptoms

Nerve damage is another possible side effect of carpal tunnel release surgery, which may cause symptoms to intensify or loss of feeling and function in the hand and fingers. Nerve damage may result from a variety of circumstances, including the surgical method utilized, the existence of underlying nerve compression or injury, and individual differences in anatomy and physiology.

To reduce the danger of nerve injury, surgeons use precise procedures and meticulous dissection to detect and preserve the median nerve that passes through the carpal tunnel. In rare circumstances, intraoperative nerve monitoring may be used to evaluate nerve function and integrity during the surgery. This helps the surgical team to make necessary modifications to avoid nerve harm.

Despite these safeguards, nerve injury is still possible in rare circumstances. Patients should be aware of the signs and symptoms of nerve damage, which include numbness, tingling, weakness, and loss of feeling in their hands and fingers. Any new or worsening symptoms should be reported to a medical professional for examination and treatment.

Scar Tissue Formation And Stiffness

Scar tissue development and stiffness are significant concerns after carpal tunnel release surgery. As the incision heals, scar tissue may develop around the surgical site, causing stiffness and reduced range of motion in the wrist and hand.

To reduce the production of excessive scar tissue, patients are often recommended to practice a modest range of motion and stretching exercises as prescribed by their doctor. This promotes healing and prevents stiffness in the afflicted region.

In rare circumstances, scar tissue growth and stiffness may need further therapies such as physical or occupational therapy. These treatments use focused exercises and procedures to improve flexibility, strength, and function in the hands and wrists.

Addressing Concerns With The Healthcare Team

If you have any worries or questions concerning carpal tunnel release surgery, you should talk honestly with your healthcare team. Your surgeon and other members of the healthcare team are there to assist you during the surgical procedure and may give information, direction, and reassurance as necessary.

Before having surgery, share any concerns or questions you may have with your surgeon. This might include inquiries regarding the treatment itself, possible risks and consequences, anticipated results, and postoperative care and recovery.

If you suffer any unexpected symptoms or difficulties throughout your recuperation, contact your healthcare professional right away. Prompt communication enables the healthcare team to quickly address issues and offer appropriate treatment and support as required.

Working closely with your healthcare team and remaining educated about the possible risks and consequences of carpal tunnel release surgery allows you to play an active part in your treatment and promotes a positive result.

CHAPTER 9

Long-Term Treatment Of Carpal Tunnel Syndrome

Monitoring For Recurrence Of Symptoms

Following carpal tunnel release surgery, it is critical to check for any symptoms of symptom recurrence. While the treatment is intended to relieve pressure on the median nerve, some circumstances may lead to symptoms recurring over time.

Pay particular attention to any recurrent symptoms, such as numbness, tingling, or weakness in the hand and fingers, to help detect recurrence. These symptoms might signal that the median nerve is once again constricted inside the carpal tunnel. Observe any changes in hand strength or coordination that might indicate a return of carpal tunnel syndrome.

Regular follow-up sessions with your healthcare practitioner are required to check your healing progress. During these meetings, your doctor will review your symptoms and may do testing, such as nerve conduction studies, to determine the function of the median nerve. These examinations may assist detect any early indicators of symptom recurrence, allowing relevant therapies to be administered as soon as possible.

In certain circumstances, lifestyle or work-related variables may lead to the recurrence of carpal tunnel syndrome symptoms. You may assist lessen the chance of recurrent symptoms by being attentive to your hand and wrist motions and avoiding activities that strain the wrist. Furthermore, making ergonomic changes to your workspace or everyday activities may assist relieve pressure on the median nerve and avoid symptom recurrence.

Strategies To Avoid Future Wrist Problems

Preventing future wrist disorders is critical for preserving long-term hand health after carpal tunnel release surgery. Implementing techniques to decrease wrist strain and promote appropriate wrist alignment may help avoid the onset of problems like repetitive strain injuries or arthritis.

One useful method is to use optimal ergonomics at work and in everyday activities. This involves keeping the wrists in neutral postures, utilizing ergonomic tools and equipment, and taking frequent pauses to relax and extend the hands and wrists. By optimizing your workstation layout and adopting appropriate ergonomics, you may lessen the pressure on your wrists and the likelihood of developing future wrist issues.

Regular exercise and strengthening of the muscles around the wrist and hand might also assist in avoiding future wrist disorders. Wrist curls, grip exercises, and stretches may help improve wrist stability and flexibility, lowering the risk of injury or strain. Incorporating these exercises into your everyday regimen will help you maintain proper hand and wrist function over time.

Lifestyle Changes For Hand Health

Making lifestyle changes to improve hand health is critical for treating carpal tunnel syndrome and avoiding future wrist issues. These adjustments may include changes to everyday activities, habits, and routines that decrease hand and wrist strain and increase overall hand well-being.

One key lifestyle change is to maintain correct hand and wrist posture when typing, writing, and using portable devices. Maintaining neutral wrist postures and avoiding excessive bending or twisting of the wrists may assist minimize strain and lower the likelihood of developing carpal tunnel syndrome or other wrist disorders.

Another lifestyle improvement is to take frequent pauses from tasks that require repetitive hand and wrist motions. Prolonged or repeated usage of the hands and wrists may lead to overuse problems like tendinitis or carpal tunnel syndrome. Taking pauses to relax and stretch the hands and wrists regularly may help avoid overuse injuries and improve hand health.

When Should I Seek Medical Attention For New Symptoms

Knowing when to seek medical assistance for new symptoms is critical to controlling carpal tunnel syndrome and avoiding complications. While some soreness or moderate symptoms may be anticipated throughout the healing time after carpal tunnel release surgery, some signs and symptoms need immediate medical attention.

If you have severe or increasing pain, numbness, tingling, or weakness in your hand or fingers, get medical assistance immediately. These symptoms might signal consequences like nerve injury or infection, necessitating prompt medical attention.

Furthermore, if you observe any changes in the look or function of your hand or wrist, such as swelling, redness, or trouble moving the fingers, you should check with your doctor. These symptoms may signal underlying problems that require more investigation and treatment.

Overall, believe your instincts and seek medical assistance if you have any concerns or queries regarding your symptoms or healing process. Your healthcare practitioner can evaluate your situation, provide appropriate therapy, and help you get the best possible results from carpal tunnel release surgery.

CHAPTER 10

Lifestyle Modifications And Preventative Measures

Ergonomic Workspace Setup

Creating an ergonomic workstation is critical for avoiding carpal tunnel syndrome (CTS) and guaranteeing comfort and efficiency at work. Begin by positioning your workstation and chair at the proper height to maintain a neutral wrist posture when typing or using a mouse. To reduce tension on the median nerve, keep your wrists straight rather than twisted up and down.

Invest in an ergonomic keyboard and mouse that supports natural hand postures and allows for free wrist mobility. Position your keyboard and mouse near your body to avoid straining your wrists and shoulders.

Consider utilizing a wrist rest to help support your wrists when you type or use a mouse. However, make sure it is not too high or too forceful since this might put further strain on the carpal tunnel.

Also, take pauses throughout the day to stretch and relax your hands and wrists. Stand up, walk about, and do some mild wrist stretches to relieve stress and avoid stiffness.

Hand And Wrist Exercises For Prevention

Regular hand and wrist exercises may help strengthen the muscles and tendons in your hands and wrists, lowering the likelihood of developing carpal tunnel syndrome. Add these exercises to your regular regimen to keep your hands and wrists supple and healthy.

Begin with wrist flexor and extensor exercises, holding each for 15-30 seconds and repeating 2-3 times on each side. These exercises serve to increase flexibility and alleviate stress in the wrist and forearm muscles.

Next, practice wrist rotations by gently rotating your wrists in circles, first clockwise, then counterclockwise. Aim for 10-15 rotations in each direction to increase joint mobility and decrease stiffness.

Hand strengthening activities, such as squeezing a stress ball or utilizing a grip strengthener, may also help prevent CTS by improving the strength and endurance of the muscles in your hands and fingers.

Identifying Early Symptoms

It is critical to detect the early signs of carpal tunnel syndrome so that you can take steps to avoid future harm. Common symptoms include numbness, tingling, and burning sensations in the thumb, index, and middle fingers, as well as weakness and clumsiness.

Pay close attention to any discomfort or soreness in your hands and wrists, particularly during tasks that demand repeated hand motions or extended wrist flexion. If you notice any of these symptoms, take a break, rest your hands, and do some mild stretches to reduce pressure on the median nerve.

Importance Of Regular Check-Ups

Regular check-ups with a healthcare practitioner are essential for tracking your hand and wrist health and detecting early indications of carpal tunnel syndrome. During periodic check-ups, your doctor may evaluate your symptoms, do diagnostic tests, and offer suitable treatments to avoid future nerve damage.

Be proactive in arranging frequent check-ups, particularly if you work in a field that requires repeated hand motions or prolonged wrist flexion. Early identification and management are critical for controlling carpal tunnel syndrome and avoiding long-term consequences.

To avoid carpal tunnel syndrome and preserve optimum hand and wrist health, use ergonomic workstation setups, and hand and wrist workouts, recognize early symptoms, and attend frequent check-ups.

Conclusion

Finally, patients, doctors, and caretakers all benefit from a thorough knowledge of carpal tunnel release (CTR) surgery. CTR is an important treatment option for those suffering from carpal tunnel syndrome (CTS), a condition that may considerably affect daily functionality and quality of life.

The choice to undergo CTR should be based on a comprehensive evaluation of the severity of symptoms, the success of conservative therapies, and the individual's general health and lifestyle. While CTR is typically safe and successful, there are certain risks and consequences to consider. As a result, patients must have open and frank talks with their healthcare professionals about the advantages and dangers of surgery before continuing with it.

For patients receiving CTR, thorough preoperative preparation and subsequent care are critical. This involves comprehending the surgical technique, managing recovery and rehabilitation goals, and following postoperative activity and treatment requirements. With strict following to these regimens, many patients may enjoy considerable alleviation from their symptoms and restore function in the afflicted hand.

Furthermore, current research and developments in surgical methods enhance and improve the results of CTR treatments. Minimally invasive treatments, including endoscopic and ultrasound-guided procedures, have the potential to minimize postoperative discomfort, speed up recovery, and enhance esthetic results. As these procedures become more extensively used, they may improve overall patient experience and satisfaction with CTR surgery.

Furthermore, maximizing patient outcomes requires a multidisciplinary approach to CTS care, which includes coordination among orthopedic surgeons, neurologists, physiotherapists, and occupational therapists.

By addressing the underlying biomechanical, neurological, and functional elements of the problem, healthcare practitioners may design treatment programs to each patient's specific requirements and encourage long-term success after CTR surgery.

Although carpal tunnel release surgery is a standard therapy for carpal tunnel syndrome, it is not a one-size-fits-all approach. Patients and healthcare professionals must collaborate to make educated choices regarding the timing and approach to surgery, as well as to guarantee thorough preoperative and postoperative care. Individuals may realize significant improvements in symptoms and function, allowing them to continue their everyday activities with more ease and confidence.

THE END